The CBCT® for Healthcare Providers

# Implementation Guide

## Bringing Compassion Training into Healthcare Systems

Center for Contemplative
Science and Compassion-Based Ethics
Emory University

Published by Center for Contemplative Science and
Compassion-Based Ethics, Emory University

1st Edition

ISBN: 978-1-962972-15-4 (Paperback edition)

# Contents

# Introduction

Compassion is core to the practice of medicine. Providing competent, kind, and compassionate healthcare requires a wide range of soft skills and humanistic qualities, in addition to technical expertise and medical knowledge. These skills need to be developed with education and training.

Students join medical school with a deep sense of purpose and meaning, and an altruistic aspiration to make a difference in people's lives. They understand that the practice of medicine is compassion in action. But during their training, they are exposed to the cynicism and indifference that are so pervasive in healthcare, and their empathy declines over time.[1] They then enter the healthcare workforce, where depression, burnout, imposter syndrome, and suicide are prevalent,[2] as are bullying and violence,[3] all of which have manifold consequences, not the least of which being their impact on patient safety.[4] Genuine and caring connections have a positive effect on the safety of both patients and providers.[5] For all these reasons, we posit that compassion training cannot be considered a mere desirable or a luxury in healthcare; it must be integrated throughout the system.

This guide offers a strategic methodology for implementing such a compassionate approach, as well as practical information for healthcare systems and schools interested in developing such an approach. CBCT® (Cognitively Based Compassion Training) for Healthcare Providers is a research-based program that aims to enhance wellbeing by cultivating resilience and compassion. It is designed to help reduce providers' physical and emotional symptoms of burnout and imposter syndrome, and increase job retention, while positively impacting patients' clinical outcomes and contributing to a greater sense of connection and meaning in the workplace. Importantly, CBCT for Healthcare Providers fosters a culture of inclusiveness and appreciation where everyone feels supported, valued, motivated, and inspired by a shared aspiration to provide quality, kind, and compassionate patient care.

Given the high demands, competitiveness, and limited resources of healthcare systems and schools, investing time and money into staff and student wellbeing can seem misplaced. However, research studies have shown that compassion improves the wellbeing of healthcare providers,

*"Compassion is essential for survival. Without cooperation, trust, gratitude, and reciprocity—as well as the many other qualities associated with compassion— humans would not have survived, let alone flourished."*

— Dacher Keltner, *Born to Be Good: The Science of a Meaningful Life*, 2009

1

positively impacts the clinical outcome of patients, and financially bene-fits healthcare systems.[6]

This implementation guide is designed to support the integration of CBCT for Healthcare Providers into healthcare education, clinics, hos-pitals, and healthcare systems. The implementation process outlined in this guide involves a thoughtful approach designed to deepen the under-standing of each organization's needs and readiness for this compassion training program, explore the best way to offer the training to different community members, and integrate the practices and skills into existing structures to contribute to long-term benefits.

Through the development of a deliberative and thoughtful plan, and a commitment over time to executing it, CBCT for Healthcare Providers can be implemented in a manner that contributes to a more caring healthcare culture, enhances the wellbeing and effectiveness of providers and staff, improves patients' outcomes, and helps the system prosper.

# Program Overview

CBCT, a program of Emory University's Center for Contemplative Science and Compassion-Based Ethics (colloquially, the Compassion Center), is a comprehensive and research-based compassion training protocol.[7] Professor Lobsang Tenzin Negi, PhD, developed CBCT in 2004, drawing from the ancient Indo-Tibetan Buddhist teachings of *lojong* along with complementary insights from emotion science to create this multilayered and practical approach.

As the most researched compassion training program of its kind, CBCT has contributed to a growing body of research linking compassion training to greater resilience and well-being. Studies suggest that compassion training not only lowers stress hormones and strengthens immune response, but also decreases rumination, activates pleasure circuits in the brain, increases self-reported happiness, fosters more optimistic and supportive communication styles, and serves as an antidote to burnout. CBCT has had a transformative impact on educators, healthcare providers, spiritual health practitioners, military veterans with post-traumatic stress disorder, adolescents in foster care, parents of children with autism, transgender youth and their parents, breast cancer survivors, and many others.[8]

Professor Negi developed CBCT in response to a plea from an undergraduate student at Emory who was committed to supporting her campus community amidst a mental health crisis. When taking a course taught by Professor Negi, she found that the practices he presented, on cultivating resilience and self-compassion and enhancing a sense of belonging and warm-hearted connection to others, could be just what her fellow students needed. Her encouragement led Professor Negi to develop CBCT as a program for people of any or no faith tradition, designed to help participants cultivate inner skills and perspectives that contribute to greater flourishing.

## CBCT Research Outcomes

Significant decreases in:

- stress biomarkers and inflammatory response[9]
- depression[10]
- loneliness[11]
- PTSD symptoms[12]

Significant increases in:

- hopefulness[13]
- compassion and related neural activity[14]
- empathy and related neural activity[15]
- self-compassion[16]

For published research on the above outcomes, visit *compassion.emory.edu.*

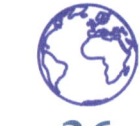

**26**
Countries Represented
by Teachers

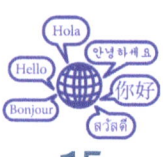

**15**
Languages

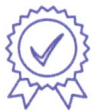

**300+**
Certified Teachers

**15**
Certified Senior
Teachers

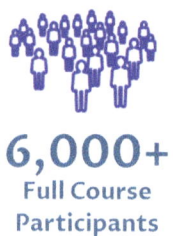

**6,000+**
Full Course
Participants

**15**
Introduced
to CBCT

## How Does CBCT Stand Out From Other Programs?

▶ CBCT holds the distinction of being one of the longest-running and most studied compassion protocols of its kind.

▶ CBCT is linked to improvements in health and wellbeing across studies.

▶ Rather than a one-size-fits-all approach, CBCT has been tailored to various sectors, including education, healthcare, and business, and for mental health practitioners, by experts in their respective fields—all with impressive results.

▶ As of 2024, CBCT has directly impacted over 50,000 people throughout 26 countries and in 15 languages, and these numbers continue to grow.

▶ CBCT forms the cornerstone of a strategic global initiative, the Compassion Shift®, which aims to advance a global culture of compassion.

Learn more about the Compassion Shift initiative at: *compassionshift.emory.edu.*

# CBCT for Healthcare Providers

In 2024, Emory's Compassion Center launched this uniquely tailored program—CBCT for Healthcare Providers—for professionals who provide patient care. Healthcare providers face challenges that cannot be underestimated. Time-consuming documentation, staff attrition, struggles with insurance, demands to shorten time with patients so that more can be seen in a day, instances of incivility, to mention a few. The challenges are too many, and this must be honored.

CBCT for Healthcare Providers is a compassion training program specifically aimed at enhancing the wellbeing of healthcare providers. It offers a variety of practices designed to strengthen resilience, foster meaningful connections and support a greater sense of efficacy in both professional and personal life. As providers cultivate the tools to deepen and expand compassion, this promotes a greater sense of purpose in life, a core component of wellbeing, fundamental for human flourishing.

It is important not to misconstrue CBCT as a "fixer"; CBCT for Healthcare Providers is not intended to mitigate the need to address any of the structural problems present in healthcare. Those must be addressed on their own terms.

The practices in this course lead to subtle (and sometimes not-so-subtle) changes in providers' emotional and social intelligence. The practices are designed to naturally shift small interactions—like the use of language, tone of voice, or gestures—that can make a world of difference to individual colleagues, patients, and the healthcare setting as a whole. These shifts may not all be conscious, but neuroscience tells us that we pick up on these subtle signals even unconsciously, and they can shape our levels of trust and confidence with each other. As a strong sense of safety and trust grows, this can have a tremendous impact on individual wellbeing and overall culture.

**Learn More About CBCT for Healthcare Providers**

*Training Compassion for Healthcare Providers: The Official Guide to CBCT for Healthcare Providers* (2025)

Compassion U™, the digital learning platform for all CBCT courses. For more information about the CBCT program, courses, and how to bring it to your organization, please visit: *compassionu.app*

# CBCT For
# Healthcare Providers: Core Skills

- Strategies for emotion regulation: attention deployment, self-distancing, and cognitive reappraisal.

- Non-judgmental awareness of the present moment experience: witnessing the arising and subsiding of mental experience, enabling a discerning response rather than an impulsive reaction.

- Self-compassion: embracing our limitations, struggles, and challenges as part of the human condition, while also making our strengths visible; learning and growing from these experiences; strengthening the alignment between our livelihood and our core values; deepening our sensitivity to the suffering of others; promoting self-agency and inner peace.

- Taking a systems-thinking view to recognize the many factors that contribute to an outcome, so many of which are beyond our control—we are humans, not superhumans.

- Focusing on intention and purpose rather than on an outcome that we cannot control.

- Identification with others based on our shared humanity, aspirations, and vulnerabilities: a portal to empathy.

- Tenderness and warm-heartedness toward an increasingly wider circle of people through the feelings of gratitude that result from the recognition of our interdependence.

- Transitioning from empathic distress to engaged compassion.

- Love and compassion as mere offerings, not reliant on outcomes or on reciprocity, simply anchored on the motivation to contribute to the joy and happiness of others (love), or to alleviate their suffering (compassion).

- Recognizing that while every action of love and compassion makes a difference, it may not be sufficient to ensure the attainment of a desirable outcome, but that does not detract from the motivation at the core of wise love and compassion.

- The joy of reconnecting to the original aspirations that led to a career in healthcare.

- Bringing meaning to every patient encounter.

# Compassion at the Core of Healthcare

Compassion is defined as the warm-hearted concern that unfolds when we witness the suffering of others and feel motivated to relieve it. Compassion has three components: (a) affective—the feeling of warm-heartedness, endearment, or tenderness; (b) cognitive—the ability to see or understand what someone else is going through; (c) motivational—the desire to see them free from their struggles. Aren't these three components inextricably linked to healthcare? Indeed, they are! Healthcare is an expression of compassion in action.

As research shows, compassion, like wellbeing, is a skill that can be developed through education and training.[17] Without being cultivated, compassion tends to be limited to those closest to us. Compassion training enables the widening of our circle of compassion, and CBCT for Healthcare Providers fosters the cultivation and embodiment of these skills.

Patients attest to the significance of compassion to their healing, and research shows that brief moments of genuine connection and kindness can impact patients' clinical outcomes.[18]

To mention but a few, compassionate care has been shown to improve patient safety and overall healthcare quality,[19] reduce time in the recovery room after surgery, reduce the amount of pain medication needed after surgery, and reduce hospitalization stay and readmission rates.[20]

Another impactful outcome of compassionate care can be seen in the treatment of homeless adults. They make frequent visits to emergency departments and often leave unsatisfied, resulting in recurring visits. Compassionate care has been shown to lead to a one-third reduction in the number of return visits within a month.[21]

Furthermore, mindfulness meditation practices, similar to those practiced in the initial modules of CBCT for Healthcare Providers, have been shown to reduce patients' perioperative anxiety and depression[22] and postoperative pain[23]; to effectively manage preoperative anxiety and postoperative pain in patients scheduled for elective surgery[24]; to reduce perioperative psychological and physiological stress responses, hospital stay, and consequently, overall cost to the patient.[25]

Kindness and compassion also bond members of healthcare teams together, fostering a supportive and inclusive environment where everyone feels safe and valued, connected by a shared motivation.

Importantly, compassion does not need to be an add-on that requires extra time and causes delays. Rather, it can be seamlessly integrated into healthcare in ways that benefit providers, patients, their families, and the healthcare system at large.

In February 2025, the World Health Organization (WHO) released a report entitled "Compassion and Primary Healthcare," underscoring that "compassion is not only essential to the core of primary healthcare but also serves as a catalyst for systemic change." It is therefore of paramount importance that compassion training become integral to healthcare education and systems.[26] The purpose of this guide is to provide a framework to facilitate the implementation of CBCT for Healthcare Providers across the healthcare spectrum.

## The Challenges Facing Healthcare Providers: Deciphering Burnout

Healthcare providers face a wide range of challenges that, if not skillfully managed, compromise their safety and wellbeing and, in turn, the safety and wellbeing of their patients. The repeated exposure to these challenges often leads to symptoms of burnout, depression, anxiety, imposter syndrome, suicidal ideation, and even suicide, sadly so prevalent among members of the healthcare workforce.[27] "Quiet quitting," which has been

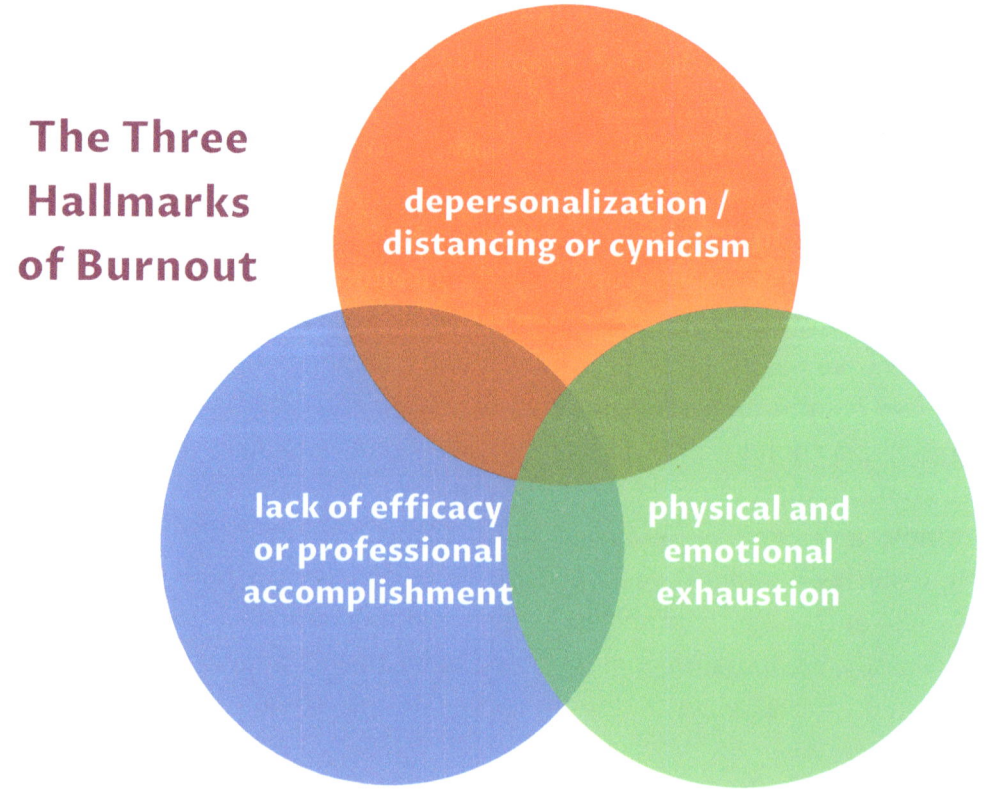

**The Three Hallmarks of Burnout**

depersonalization / distancing or cynicism

lack of efficacy or professional accomplishment

physical and emotional exhaustion

defined as "opting out of tasks beyond one's assigned duties and/or becoming less psychologically invested in work,"[28] a sign of burnout, disillusionment, and cynicism, has also become a prevalent phenomenon among healthcare professionals.[29]

Burnout has three hallmarks: depersonalization/distancing or cynicism, physical and emotional exhaustion, and lack of efficacy or professional accomplishment.[30] There is a sense of a loss of purpose accompanied by feelings of disillusionment and worthlessness, a drastic departure from the original, so often altruistic, motivation to pursue a career in healthcare.

Myriad factors contribute to burnout; hence, any attempt to single out a determining or prevailing cause will likely offer an oversimplification of a complex problem. Thus, the solution must also be comprehensive. Compassion and emotion-regulation education and training are indispensable to healthcare providers' ability to navigate these challenges with self-compassion and a sense of purpose. For this to be sustainable, the institution must foster a culture of inclusiveness and appreciation where everyone feels supported, valued, and connected by a shared aspiration to provide compassionate care to their patients and each other.

## Depersonalization, Distancing, and Cynicism

Of the three hallmarks of burnout, the core is arguably depersonalization, distancing, and cynicism. The disconnection is not only from the patient but also from the original, often altruistic, motivation that led to the career in healthcare. It is a disconnection from purpose and meaning, which are central components of our wellbeing.

There is a core contradiction in the hidden curriculum that is often taught in medical schools. While the main curriculum underscores the importance of treating the patient, not the disease, the hidden curriculum teaches students to distance themselves from their patients, presumably to protect themselves from the emotional burden of care. Research has proven this false.[31] Distancing has a negative impact not only on patients but also on physicians.[32] As discussed by Thangarasu and colleagues, "empathy can be taught, patients teach it best, and distancing makes malpractice litigations more likely to occur".[33]

The disconnection from the patient undermines the sense of reward that genuine connections may engender, while the disconnection from purpose erodes our resilience. Compassion training mitigates distancing from our patients and purpose.

## *Physical and Emotional Exhaustion*

Emotional exhaustion, the second hallmark of burnout, may result from empathy fatigue. Affective or emotional empathy, the ability to feel the joy or the suffering of others, is a transient stage in the arousal of compassion. If stationary, affective empathy can lead to emotional exhaustion and empathic distress, where the suffering of another starts to feel unbearable. Compassion training fosters the cultivation of skills that enable the transition from empathic distress to empathic concern and engaged compassion—a shift from feeling overwhelmed to feeling connected, motivated, and able to discern how we can help.

Emotional exhaustion can also arise when we forget that multiple factors contribute to an outcome, and that we lack control of many of these. Many times, when the problem cannot be fixed or a desired outcome cannot be attained, feelings of hopelessness, irritation, or even anger may arise, often resulting in turning away, "throwing the towel" in defeat. In contrast, compassion does not depend on the attainment of a desired outcome or on reciprocity to be sustained. Compassion helps us recognize that, even though we want to eradicate suffering, we simply don't have the power to make that happen every time. This is not to say that our efforts make no difference—quite the contrary.

After a physically exhausting and emotionally challenging long day at the hospital, if a desired patient outcome can't be attained, what is most needed is self-compassion, a sense of purpose, a feeling of joy and reward for the care given. This depends on the recognition that, while not capable of changing the outcome, the care that was provided did make a difference: It made the patient and their partner/family feel supported and nurtured, altogether easing the process and making all involved feel safe and cared for. Recognizing this requires many skills. In the absence of these skills, feelings of defeat, despair, and even guilt, shame, or fear may arise, particularly if an error was made.

Although self-compassion has been shown to protect against burnout, there are many misconceptions about it that, if not addressed, may become an obstacle to its practice. Some of these misconceptions include that self-compassion might lower motivation, lead to self-indulgence, or decrease the sense of personal responsibility.[34] Contrary to that, research shows that self-compassion increases self-improvement motivation,[35] promotes long-term benefits rather than short-term pleasures, and enables people to take greater personal responsibility for their actions.[36] Self-compassion is conducive to a psychophysiological response pattern of reduced arousal (reduced heart rate and skin conductance) and increased parasympathetic activation (increased heart rate variability) that is associated with effective emotion regulation in times of adversity, setting a foundation for feelings of safety and connectedness.[37]

CBCT for Healthcare Providers fosters the skills of self-compassion, compassion for others, and emotion regulation that, together, can mitigate emotional exhaustion.

## Lack of Efficacy or Professional Accomplishment

Lastly, the sense of a lack of efficacy or professional accomplishment experienced in burnout can also be mitigated with self-compassion, compassion for others, and emotion-regulation training.

Self-compassion is an important skill when it comes to combating a perceived lack of efficacy, as it helps individuals to make visible that they are not superhuman but human, with certain limitations and vulnerabilities. Self-compassion also reminds them of their strengths and of what they are doing well, instead of getting stuck only noticing those limitations or mistakes. Self-compassion helps them feel that they are not alone in failing at times, and that setbacks can become opportunities for learning and growth. Furthermore, the sense of shared humanity that arises with self-compassion practice heightens our sensitivity to others' sufferings, adversities, and vulnerabilities. With this greater understanding of others, through our enhanced connection and empathy, we can more meaningfully respond to their struggles.

Compassion for others involves seeing what someone is up against and having the warm-hearted wish to see them free from that suffering. But compassion without wisdom is like a bird with one wing: It can't fly. This wisdom, or discernment, plays the important role of uncovering the many causes and conditions that contribute to the suffering we want to alleviate. The more deeply we understand the factors at play, the better able we are to act and effect change. Discernment also allows us to see how even small actions can make a powerful impact and ripple out in ways we may not see for ourselves. Wise compassion helps us to turn our focus to what we *can* do to help instead of getting caught up in an outcome we cannot control. All of these skills are cultivated in CBCT for Healthcare Providers.

# History of CBCT Implementation in Healthcare

This section highlights several examples of CBCT implementation in various healthcare settings over the last decade, and the positive impacts CBCT has made in programs for chaplains, nurses, physicians, medical students, and others in the system.

## Emory School of Medicine

In 2014, the Emory School of Medicine invited Professor Negi to teach a comprehensive CBCT course to 20 of its top leaders, including Dean Christian Larsen, MD. This experience convinced Dean Larsen and other leaders—including Executive Dean of Education William J. Eley, MD, and Associate Dean of Students Ira Schwartz, MD—that CBCT could serve as an antidote to a number of the common struggles that plague physicians and seem to begin during their medical training, including depersonalization, depression, suicidality, and anxiety.

This interest led to Dean Larsen's funding of a randomized control trial—led by veteran CBCT researcher and medical anthropologist Jennifer Mascaro, PhD—that tailored CBCT for second-year medical students. The study's results showed a significant increase in compassion among the medical students, as well as decreases in loneliness, sleep disturbances, and depression symptoms. For more than 10 years now, Emory's Compassion Center has successfully taught CBCT to hundreds of Emory physicians and physicians-in-training, as well as to genetic counselors, physical therapists, nurses, and physician's assistants, via this partnership.

## Spiritual Health at Emory Healthcare

In 2016, another partnership bloomed between the Compassion Center and Emory Healthcare, this time with the Department of Spiritual Health.

This department oversees the hospital chaplains and houses one of the largest hospital-chaplaincy training programs in the United States. The department's leadership, especially Executive Director George Grant, PhD, and Director of Education Maureen Shelton, MDiv, had been searching for a training program that would address the emerging and changing needs for hospital chaplains—especially the real need to serve an increasingly diverse population of patients and staff who bring with them a widening variety of beliefs and traditions. They found CBCT's approach promising from the start, thanks to its emphasis on values and ethics and its alignment with many people's understandings of spirituality, while also respecting the beliefs of all major faith traditions.

At first, CBCT was folded into chaplaincy education, but soon the chaplains began to report using their CBCT practices to support active patient and staff encounters. From these insights, Compassion-Centered Spiritual Health (CCSH™) was established and soon evolved into a formal training curriculum that builds on CBCT to bolster the wellbeing, resilience, and compassion of healthcare patients and staff. This generative collaboration augments spiritual health education and best practices with CBCT. CCSH interventions are delivered by spiritual care professionals trained in both CBCT and ACPE: The Standard in Spiritual Care and Education. Emory now trains chaplains internationally and certifies them as CCSH-registered clinicians. See *ccsh.emory.edu* for more information.

## Nursing at Emory Healthcare

Since 2017, the Compassion Center has collaborated with the Emory Nursing Experience at the Nell Hodgson Woodruff School of Nursing to offer CBCT for nurses and other providers as continuing nursing education (CNE) credit.

During the Covid-19 pandemic, the School of Nursing, under the direction of research scientist Nicholas Giordano, PhD, received a workplace wellbeing grant from the National Institutes of Health to offer two programs to frontline workers in the Emory hospitals and adjacent hospital systems to address burnout and improve professional quality of life and resilience. The programs are CBCT and the Community Resilience Model (CRM), which is a shorter training that is incorporated into the first module of CBCT training. Both programs were implemented for three years. Nicknamed ARROW (Atlanta's Resilience Resources fOr Frontline Workers), the program hosted 59 training events that trained 761 healthcare providers and staff. Preliminary analysis (currently under review for publication) suggests that trainees' compassion fatigue, a key component of professional quality of life, decreased for up to three months after engaging in any programmatic offering. Nurses and other healthcare providers attending CBCT were observed to have additional declines in scores of compassion fatigue. ARROW supported 68 healthcare personnel to become either CRM- or CBCT-certified instructors via a train-the-trainer program. As of the summer of 2025, these new trainers continued to offer training opportunities to an additional 772 colleagues.

## University of Illinois College of Medicine Peoria

In 2016, a group of five faculty from the College of Medicine and one counselor from the Methodist College of Nursing pursued the CBCT Teacher Certification training offered by the Compassion Center. With this training, they intended to offer CBCT courses to medical students, residents, fellows, all members of the healthcare workforce in the affiliated hospitals, the administrative staff at the college of medicine, and the Peoria community at large. As a final requirement to attain certification, the trainees co-taught a CBCT course for the first time, under supervision. They offered four courses simultaneously, all in-person, for a total of 60 participants, evenly distributed in classes of 15 participants each. The teachers-in-training felt that it would be important for leadership to learn what CBCT entailed directly from them, certain that this would not only put to rest any misconceptions or concerns about the program they might have had, but it would also allow them to have a direct experience of the benefits of compassion training. They invited everyone who served in a leading role: the regional dean, all associate and assistant deans, the members of the C-suite of the affiliated hospitals, the heads and chairs of all departments, the superintendent of the Peoria Public School system, the mayor, and the manager of the city. With the exception of the mayor, who could not participate due to scheduling conflicts, everyone joined the program.

Enrollment was as successful as it was for two reasons. First, the regional dean at the time, Dr. Sara Rush, personally requested that all the invitees attend the course. Without such strong support from the regional dean of the college, recruitment would likely not have been as successful. Second, the teachers-in-training made every effort to avoid scheduling conflicts by offering the courses on two different days and at two different times, before and after working hours. Attendance was nearly 100 percent throughout the 8 weeks. An anonymous post-course survey strongly demonstrated everyone's engagement and appreciation, at times expressing surprise at how much they benefited from the course. This great success opened the doors for offering CBCT courses to different sectors of the healthcare ecosystem, teachers in the public school system, and even the leadership of the Peoria Police Department.

For the past several years, the CBCT-trained faculty have offered an intensive, in-person three-day CBCT course to incoming medical students, just before their school orientation week. This has proven very successful. While this course is not mandatory, a group of students always volunteers to join the training. These students develop strong ties to each other during this training and remain supportive of each other throughout the four years of medical school.

A few years after the first group of faculty became certified to teach CBCT, they were awarded an internal grant to support training additional faculty, this time to include colleagues from the other two campuses of the College of Medicine, Chicago and Rockford. They have since become certified, and CBCT is now available for students and members of the healthcare workforce in the three campuses of the University of Illinois College of Medicine.

## Sitamarhi District Hospital in India

Kartik Varma has served as a core team member of the Piramal School of Leadership since 2017, with a particular focus on systems transformation, organization development, and leadership development. His vision is that compassion needs to be embedded into every part of the healthcare system, including how jobs are defined, performances managed, leadership built, and teams led.

This vision is being successfully implemented in the Sitamarhi District Hospital, which serves 3.42 million people in one of Bihar's poorest districts. Before the implementation of CBCT, the Sitamarhi District Hospital was ranked among the worst-performing hospitals in Bihar. There was a decline in the average patient footfall per month, a deeply hierarchical culture, frequent altercations between patients and staff, and miscommunication and disagreements between team members.

The implementation of CBCT at this hospital began in 2021 with the aim of building a compassionate healthcare system in Bihar by 2030, "transforming citizen experience through CBCT for 100,000 healthcare workers." This was done by first bringing CBCT workshops to the 230 staff. Along with the workshops, workplace rules, rewards, and recognition were redesigned to support this compassionate mission. Compassion training was offered in particular to nursing staff, new medical officers, and leaders.

Since CBCT's implementation, patient footfall has increased from 9,000 to 15,000. The Sitamarhi District Hospital now ranks first in Bihar and has achieved the MusQan certification, which is the highest certificate for quality child-friendly care. It received the highest quality certificate awarded to hospitals in India (NQAS) and received multiple awards in 2023, including Best Hospital in Bihar.

Important to the success of this project was a well-trained cadre of certified CBCT instructors who worked with the hospital leadership to plan classes that fit the scheduling needs of the hospital staff. The project also benefited from starting with the buy-in of leadership. For example, though culturally it is normal for many staff to sit on the floor or stand during meetings while physicians sit in chairs, in the CBCT classes, the instructors brought floor cushions for all participants, and the physicians sat on the floor with everyone else. The instructors helped the participants connect this novel seating arrangement to the CBCT course content—in particular, the ability to see that, despite our differences, at a very important level, we are all the same. Both physicians and lower-level staff reported that this was a moving and significant part of the course that reinforced the content, helping it extend beyond the classroom and into the everyday work.

## Lessons Learned: Challenges and Opportunities

While each institution has its own culture, some lessons pertain to all. The following are the main takeaways from our collective experience regarding what is most critical for a successful CBCT implementation:

- Flexibility and adaptability

- Engaging the leadership at an early stage

- Disseminating information about CBCT to the different sectors of the organization through seminars, town hall meetings, and short workshops

- Identifying individuals interested in becoming teachers of the program and facilitating their training

- Providing a space for meditation and weekly practice sessions facilitated by a certified CBCT teacher

It is often asked whether CBCT should be offered as an optional or a mandatory course. There is no simple answer to this question because it depends on context. While the leadership must be fully committed to its implementation, that alone is insufficient. Different sectors of the organization must also be interested in implementation, and that requires time for everyone to get informed about CBCT, what it entails, and how it can benefit them, personally and professionally. And without a comprehensive strategic plan for implementation, as presented in this guide, a mandatory course is unlikely to succeed, irrespective of the organization's culture and the leadership's level of commitment. It is important to view implementation as a process that includes sequential stages reflecting increasing levels of engagement across the organization, leading toward a top-down and bottom-up shared motivation for a full implementation.

Ultimately, the motivation to join a collective effort to embed compassion into every part of the healthcare system can drive everyone in the organization to embrace the training. The pursuit of a noble cause, rooted in shared values, promotes a sense of purpose, identification with one another, and safety.

Emory University is a good example, being at an advanced stage of this process. CBCT is now being offered to chaplains, nurses, and other providers, as well as to incoming medical students as part of the main curriculum. The various synergistic partnerships that have been established with the Compassion Center have proven invaluable to the success of these implementation processes.

# A Study on CBCT for Leprosy Care Providers

*"This is the first time in 35 years that I, as a female cleaner, am treated the same as the civil surgeon."*

— Staff member of Sitamarhi District Hospital

Leprosy is a curable disease, and for several decades, the medicine and science have been available to eradicate its spread without requiring the isolation of patients. Major progress by global health institutions has reduced the number of leprosy cases to under 250,000 worldwide. Despite this, leprosy remains a disease that still carries a heavy burden of stigma, especially in parts of the world where it remains prevalent. This stigma often leads to people avoiding treatment and feeling isolated or dehumanized. Unfortunately, even healthcare workers can sometimes hold negative attitudes, affecting patients' quality of care. Experts in the field have identified stigma as one of the primary impediments to the full eradication of the disease.

A grant from No Leprosy Remains (NLR) International was awarded to the Taskforce for Global Health and Emory University's Compassion Center to tailor CBCT to address this stigma by helping healthcare workers better understand leprosy and respond to the patients' needs with greater compassion and reduced judgment.

The initial study was set in public health clinics in Jharkhand, one of India's states with high levels of poverty and leprosy, which are often related. The initial intervention was offered to 80 healthcare workers, a combination of physicians and paramedical technicians who commonly treat persons living with leprosy. Researchers began by collecting information through surveys and interviews to understand how stigma and compassion were experienced and expressed. They found that many patients felt stigmatized and that their overall wellbeing was lower, especially among older individuals and those with more severe forms of the disease. Among healthcare workers, those with more experience and prior training in leprosy care tended to show more compassion and less social distance from patients.

Based on these findings, leaders at the Compassion Center worked with certified teachers at the Piramal Foundation, an India-based organization that already had experience bringing compassion training to distressed healthcare settings (see case study of Sitamarhi hospital on page 15), to create a tailored CBCT program for leprosy care providers. The tailoring, based on insights from initial surveys by the study team, was designed to offer the full CBCT course, while emphasizing the aspects of the training that will aid healthcare workers in becoming more aware of the stigma their patients face, less susceptible to their conditioned distancing and stigmatizing behaviors toward these patients, and thus more able to respond connect with patients as individuals, leading to more compassionate care.

In one touching anecdote from the initial study, a physician recalled that, after the CBCT training, he met with a patient who explained that they had symptoms that indicated leprosy. The physician noted that he reflexively stepped away from the patient slightly at this news. But upon noticing this behavior, he recalled that this reflex was based on biases learned from his upbringing, not his medical training. Recalling that leprosy cannot be transmitted through proximity, he was able to look the patient in the eye, connect to them as a person, and step closer to continue the evaluation. The physician reported that he was sure that this new way of relating, along with helping him stay true to his intentions and values as a caregiver, was reassuring for the patient and allowed the patient to better receive the diagnosis and to hear and follow the treatment instructions. The physician felt that the chances of successful treatment were significantly higher given this shift in the relationship.

The initial CBCT for Leprosy Care Providers training was rolled out in 2025, and the research team collected anecdotal evidence of acceptability within the target population. Follow-up studies are planned. The program is poised to create a more respectful and supportive healthcare environment, where people affected by leprosy feel seen, valued, and cared for—not just medically, but as whole human beings. This improved quality of care should lead to greater comprehension of and adherence to treatments that, if applied more universally, may support the eventual eradication of leprosy from the human experience.

# Implementation Process

A cohesive plan for implementing CBCT for Healthcare Providers in healthcare education, clinics, and hospitals goes beyond offering a single training or workshop. Sustainable implementation involves a thoughtful approach to bringing CBCT to each healthcare system in a way that meets its specific needs and allows for opportunities for the approach to be integrated in culturally meaningful ways. This section walks through a process for implementing CBCT for Healthcare Providers in various healthcare settings.

## The Four Components
### of CBCT for Healthcare Providers Implementation

| | | | |
|---|---|---|---|
| **1** | | **Set the Foundation** | Lay the groundwork for the implementation of CBCT for Healthcare Providers. |
| **2** | | **Engage the Community** | Introduce CBCT for Healthcare Providers to the organization through orientation sessions to create buy-in, appoint CBCT ambassadors, and develop plans for implementation. |
| **3** | | **Implement the Training** | Deliver CBCT for Healthcare Providers training. |
| **4** | | **Support Ongoing Integration** | Sustain, develop, and continuously integrate CBCT for Healthcare Providers. |

# Component 1
## Set the Foundation

| | | | |
|---|---|---|---|
| **1** | **Set the Foundation**<br><br>Lay the groundwork for the implementation of CBCT for Healthcare Providers. | | **Engage Goals and Vision** |
| | | | **Engage the Leadership** |
| | | | **Consider Needs and Readiness** |

 ## Establish Goals and Vision

The process starts with a clear vision, followed by a strategic plan detailing a path, a timeline with sequential goals and milestones, an assessment of cost, and the development of a budget for implementation and sustainability of the program in the organization, with periodic assessments to monitor effectiveness over time.

The vision should be constructive rather than reactive, a vision for a culture where compassion is embedded into every part of the healthcare system, a vision that entices everyone to embrace it and to feel pride at being a member of the institution. The positive impacts on wellbeing and the many indicators mentioned earlier represent byproducts of a genuinely kind and compassionate culture. It is important to reflect on the following questions before implementing CBCT for Healthcare Providers. Through thoughtful consideration of these questions, the goals and vision of implementation can be established.

| *Guiding Questions – Establish Goals and Vision* | What does CBCT for Healthcare Providers have to offer this setting? What are the needs we are addressing and/or the opportunities we see? |
| --- | --- |
| | What are the main goals and desired outcomes of implementing CBCT for Healthcare Providers? Are there specific changes that we hope implementation would lead to? |
| | How can CBCT be integrated into existing employee wellbeing offerings and/or institutional structures to support individual and organizational flourishing? |
| | How does the implementation of CBCT for Healthcare Providers fit into the organization's vision? How does this work align with our values and culture? |

 ## Engage the Leadership

The leadership needs to be shown the scientific evidence behind CBCT and the positive impact of compassion training on provider wellbeing, patient clinical outcomes and satisfaction, and the healthcare system's financial success. However, compassion training cannot be transactional. There needs to be a connection to the value of compassion, a genuine desire to instill a compassionate culture that manifests at all levels of the system, and an understanding that the positive impacts on many indicators of success are natural byproducts.

While the system may have its prevailing culture, each sector within the organization and each specialty in medicine has its own unique culture. All of these must be honored and taken into consideration during the implementation process. Each culture or microculture develops within certain contexts and because of numerous factors, with the values and actions of leaders being chief among them. Thus, it is important to hear from the various leaders across the system to understand each culture, so that aspects of the implementation process may be tailored to best suit their needs and context. It is also important to emphasize that this process cannot stop at the level of leadership. Everyone needs to feel that their voices are heard and that they are being valued. This requires time to listen and learn, not through surveys, but through heart-to-heart conversations and connections.

 ## Consider Needs and Readiness

Determining each sector's readiness for CBCT implementation is essential. This involves reflecting on the current climate and conditions for implementation, including capacity, resources, assets, and needs. This process builds on the vision and goal-setting reflection to support leaders in making decisions about CBCT training options and implementation structures.

*Guiding Questions – Consider Needs and Readiness*

What would support, improve, and/or sustain the current culture and climate? What is working well, and where are areas of concern?

What is already in place (wellness programming, healthcare initiatives, team-building activities, staff appreciation events, etc.) that can build upon and support this work?

What is the composition (seniority, skill level, geographical reach, etc.) of the organization's employees and other stakeholders? What service duration patterns are there? Is there high staff turnover, or do employees tend to stay for a number of years?

When (if ever) is professional development time offered, and how can this time best be used to meet employee and organizational needs?

What financial, human, and physical resources are available, and how can these be used to plan and support the training and implementation of CBCT?

What does our organization have the capacity to commit to? What will be needed to sustain the work of CBCT implementation?

Who might be the early adopters of CBCT for Healthcare Providers (individuals or groups who may already be interested or would be more likely to express interest)?

Who are the organization's disproportionate influencers? Are there any skeptics or detractors who would benefit from additional focus?

What external resources (speakers, peer organizations, CBCT teachers and materials, etc.) are available?

# Component 2
## Engage Community

### 2 — Engage the Organization

Introduce CBCT for Healthcare Providers to the organization through orientation sessions to create buy-in, appoint CBCT ambassadors, and develop plans for implementation.

- Identify All-Inclusive Teams
- Offer an Orientation Session
- Appoint CBCT Ambassadors
- Develop a Stakeholder Management Plan
- Develop and Execute a Communication Plan

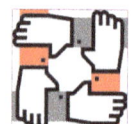

### Identify All-Inclusive Teams

Engaging members of the organization in the implementation process needs to be all-inclusive because everyone matters and every patient encounter makes a difference. Janitors, patient transporters, those at the reception desk, those who answer calls to schedule appointments—everyone needs to be part of the process.

Irrespective of the organization's size, we are most affected by the quality of the interactions with our direct co-workers. The dynamics of each group or team—each cell—is unique and needs to be understood. When planning to engage members of the organization, identify each cell so that they may be grouped. This will allow for implementation that caters to the needs of each cell rather than adopting a one-size-fits-all approach. Such cells often include supporting staff, nurses, physical therapists, speech therapists, physician assistants, physicians, surgeons, etc.

 ## Offer an Orientation Session

Community members need to be introduced to CBCT for Healthcare Providers, not through a lecture delivered to a large audience, but through small group sessions that promote sharing of ideas and addressing misconceptions. This will also help to identify anyone who might be natural ambassadors for the program and play a pivotal role in sustaining it post-implementation.

Sessions should include members of the healthcare workforce that work together, as part of a team, or a small division. This is important because, as discussed before, each team/division has its own culture and struggles. An important byproduct of CBCT for Healthcare Providers is the strengthening of connections and improvement of relationships.

A patient-centered approach may be utilized to assemble these small groups so that everyone who is directly or indirectly involved in the care of the patients in each ward, clinic, or sector would remain together as a group throughout the sessions.

In preparation for these sessions, invite participants to imagine what it would be like if compassion were embedded in every part of the healthcare system, to think what might be necessary to make that happen, and to discern how each member of the community might contribute to making this vision a reality. What is in their collective reach? Their reflections can then be shared in the small group session.

The vision for a compassionate healthcare system and a brief overview of CBCT for Healthcare Providers (listing key scientific findings supporting its benefits) should be made available at the end of the session. This could be done by providing sections from the Introduction and Program Overview sections of this guide, sharing orientation session slides, or developing new materials that contain this information.

## *Orientation Session Content*

**Note:** *For a more in-depth overview that includes reflective and interactive practices, a certified CBCT teacher is required to facilitate the session. See "Introductory Offerings" on page 35 for more information.*

### An Overview of CBCT for Healthcare Providers (~15 min)

This section will briefly introduce the system's vision for a transformative culture of compassion and present an overview of CBCT for Healthcare Providers, outlining the framework and background of CBCT, its benefits for participants, its approach to cultivating resilience and wellbeing, and the science that supports it. This brief overview should be facilitated by a senior member of the implementation team. It will establish how CBCT will foster implementation of the vision.

### The Implementation Process (~30 min)

This section goes over the goals of implementation, options for implementation, possible next steps, and community engagement possibilities. When describing this process, the facilitator should:

- Articulate a clear alignment to existing organizational vision and strategy and a clear rationale for choosing to implement CBCT.

- Be authentic about your personal investment in CBCT.

- Make connections between CBCT and other wellbeing initiatives that might already be part of the organizational culture.

- Highlight how CBCT stands out. What makes CBCT different? Discuss the challenges and opportunities that may arise from this work.

- Acknowledge, if appropriate, the possibility of change fatigue in the organization.

### Discussion, Collaboration, and Further Communication (~15 minutes)

Lastly, the facilitator should field questions and hear from session participants about ideas, areas for further consideration, and any concerns. In preparation for this discussion, the facilitator will lead the group in the co-creation of guiding principles that will make them feel safe, heard, not judged, etc.

The content and outcomes of the orientation session can be made available to the whole organization via communication channels, as appropriate.

## Appoint CBCT Ambassadors

During the small group orientation sessions, it often becomes evident who seems most genuinely engaged and enthusiastic. These individuals can then be invited to serve as CBCT ambassadors. Importantly, the organization's leadership should not be exempted. To have a CBCT ambassador on the leadership team is very important not only for the sustainability of the new culture of compassion, but also as evidence of leadership's commitment to a culture of compassion across the system.

No one should feel obliged to accept the invitation. It must be voluntary and driven by a genuine interest. If nobody in the group stands out as being distinctively engaged, a general request for volunteer participation as a program ambassador can be made. If no member of the group volunteers, an ambassador from another group may be asked to assist.

---

### Encouraging CBCT Ambassadors to Become Certified CBCT Teachers

▶ Offer regular CBCT for Healthcare Providers courses. This is a prerequisite for the CBCT Teacher Certification program.

▶ Share the following information about the CBCT Teacher Certification program:

- Opportunities and benefits of certification:
  - Ability to teach CBCT to fellow healthcare workers (in their organization and beyond), and to members of the general public
  - Access to a global compassion community of other certified CBCT instructors (healthcare workers and individuals in other sectors)
  - Deepened familiarity with the content and practices of CBCT and enhanced personal wellbeing
- Funding and scholarship opportunities available (if applicable)
- Certification process details (visit *compassionu.app/teacher-certification* for this information)

---

# The Role of CBCT Ambassadors

## Support the implementation process.

- Organize the first CBCT for Healthcare Providers course with early adopters.

- Make a plan to roll out the course to different groups in the organization.

- Support the sustainability of the program.

## Teach CBCT for Healthcare Providers courses and community practice sessions to peers (for the ambassadors that choose to go through CBCT Teacher Certification).

- To sustain a culture of compassion, it is important to certify ambassadors to teach CBCT in the organization. Participation in this should be voluntary. Ambassadors who choose this path will participate in the CBCT Teacher Certification program.

- Facilitate weekly community practice sessions to promote the sustainability of the skills cultivated during the training (described further on page 43).

- Offer courses and introductory sessions to the small groups and teams that were identified in the first phase of the implementation process. These offerings are described in Component 3: Implement the Training.

## Liaise with the research and assessment team.

- Publish any scientific reports coming out of the research and assessment team in high visibility peer-reviewed journals to inspire other systems and organizations to implement the vision for truly compassionate healthcare.

**Note:** research and assessment teams should ideally not be part of the organization, to ensure transparency and unbiased analyses.

## Meet regularly to debrief and plan.

- Share experiences leading respective sessions.

- Address any challenges that may have arisen and explore opportunities.

- Facilitate integration across units and divisions.

- Plan and promote events and initiatives—including a lecture series featuring guest speakers to present current advancements on contemplative science and compassion in healthcare.

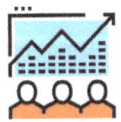

# Develop a Stakeholder Management Plan

## Conduct a Stakeholder Audit

In Component 1: Set the Foundation, the needs and readiness of the healthcare system were considered. Given that each specialty and healthcare team has its own culture, they all need to be heard and understood. With this information, the CBCT ambassadors can now assess the needs and readiness of a broader network of organizational stakeholders. It should be underscored, however, that at least one member of the leadership must be a CBCT ambassador. This process allows for greater understanding of all voices within the system, including those of stakeholders, thus facilitating an implementation strategy that is fully aligned with the vision, culturally sensitive, and maximally responsive. While optional, repeating this process can be beneficial, as it allows the organization to better understand stakeholders' perspectives, thus supporting CBCT's successful implementation.

## Develop a Stakeholder Plan

Using input from the audit, use stakeholder mapping tools to identify stakeholder risks and opportunities, and then develop a detailed relationship management plan to address these. This plan will require clear prioritization of areas to address and should be strongly linked to the overall communications plan.

## Monitor and Adjust

Stakeholder engagement can be monitored through a variety of methods, depending on which is most suitable for the organization. Interviews, surveys, focus groups, and feedback are all useful methods. The CBCT ambassadors should review the outputs of these methods and adjust their stakeholder relationship management accordingly.

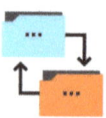 # Develop and Execute a Communication Plan

The CBCT ambassadors should work together to develop a communication plan. The purpose of communication related to CBCT for Healthcare Providers is to inform and engage employees about why CBCT is being implemented, what they can expect from CBCT, and how they can get involved in CBCT. First and foremost, however, the communication plan should be centered around the vision to embed compassion in every part of the system, explaining how CBCT may be conducive to the attainment of this vision.

## Communication Plan Goals

- Gaining support from organization employees
- Sparking interest in different stakeholder groups
- Developing relationships to allow for questions about and exploration of CBCT
- Sharing information about different CBCT offerings and practices
- Keeping people engaged and excited about CBCT practices and training experiences
- Providing support for initial and ongoing CBCT integration

# Component 3
## Implement the Training

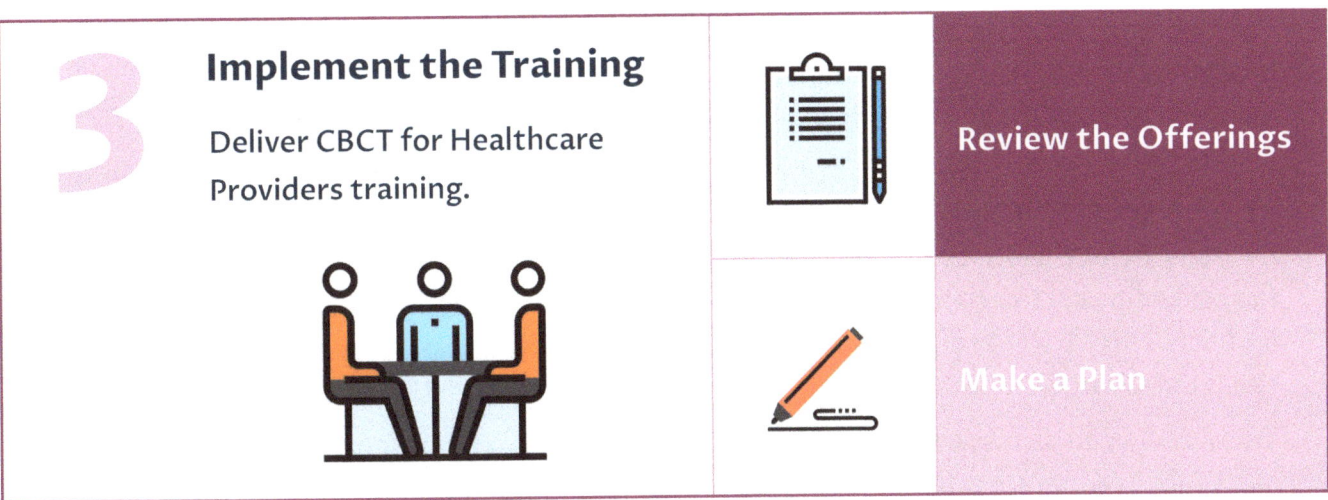

**Implement the Training**

Deliver CBCT for Healthcare Providers training.

**Review the Offerings**

**Make a Plan**

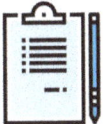 ## Review the Offerings

Training Compassion for Healthcare Providers is the full CBCT for Healthcare Providers course. This is a 10-week course accessible through Compassion U, a digital learning platform that comprises the entirety of the CBCT program, tailored for healthcare professionals, and includes live hour-long weekly sessions facilitated by one or two certified CBCT instructors. This is the most comprehensive training modality.

Training Compassion for Healthcare Providers encompasses 10 self-guided learning experiences: Overview, Modules 1–8, and What's Next. Participants are expected to learn the content and complete each module's insight activities and meditation practices at their preferred time, in advance of the weekly live sessions.

Once certified to facilitate Compassion U sessions, any of the CBCT ambassadors may lead or co-lead these sessions.

## Training Compassion for Healthcare Providers

### Training Compassion for Healthcare Providers (16–24 hours)

**Brief Description:** A deep dive into the eight CBCT modules, tailored for those who work in healthcare organizations. Each module introduces new content, reflective exercises, and practices designed to strengthen inner skills and insights and support their application into everyday life.

The Training Compassion for Healthcare Providers course is offered through Compassion U, a user-friendly app that delivers CBCT course content and provides access to instructional videos, activities, practices, and a compassion community, among other resources.

Courses include live sessions with other participants, facilitated by certified CBCT teachers. These live sessions are typically one hour each and occur weekly over nine weeks. Prior to each live session, participants engage in the self-guided content, activities, and practices on Compassion U.

This course can also serve as a prerequisite for those who are interested in applying for the CBCT Teacher Certification program.

**Format:**

- Self-guided on digital learning platform, Compassion U (8–16 hours, typically 1.5 hours per week)

- Live sessions in person or via videoconference, facilitated by a certified CBCT teacher (9 hours of live sessions, typically 1 hour per week)

## Introductory Offerings

### Overview of Training Compassion for Healthcare Providers (30 minutes–1.5 hours)

**Brief Description:** The Overview offered in the Training Compassion for Healthcare Providers course on Compassion U is a self-guided experience that orients participants to the content and practices of the course, introduces compassion and compassion training, and includes reflective exercises and practices that set a foundation for the course and give a glimpse into the types of experiences that participants will engage in throughout the rest of the course. The Overview is a free experience available to anyone through Compassion U.

**Format:**
- Fully self-guided on digital learning platform, Compassion U

### Introduction to CBCT – Seminar (45 minutes–3 hours)

**Brief Description:** An introduction to CBCT, including a sample practice or two. This training provides an overview of CBCT, including an exploration of the framework and its history, its benefits for employees and leaders, its approach to cultivating resilience and wellbeing, and the science that supports it.

**Format:**
- Live session in person or via videoconference, facilitated by a certified CBCT teacher

### A Taste of CBCT – Workshop (4–8 hours)

**Brief Description:** This training exposes participants to the key themes, skills, and insights of the CBCT course, and introduces some of the reflective exercises and informal and formal practices. This workshop provides a taste of the CBCT experience, allowing individuals to begin exploring and strengthening the capacities related to resilience and compassion before diving into the training. This could be done in one long session or broken up into several shorter sessions over multiple days.

**Format:**
- Live session(s) in person or via videoconference, facilitated by a certified CBCT teacher

# Make a Plan

**Want to Bring CBCT to Your Organization?**

Visit *compassionu. app/ for-organizations*

The path for CBCT for Healthcare Providers training will vary, depending on the organization's specific needs and structure. For example, if you begin by offering CBCT for Healthcare Providers to a group already on board with the idea of the program, they may dive straight into the training, meeting weekly over nine weeks. If there is a group that has less time and/or buy-in, they may begin with one of the introductory offerings. When making a plan to offer CBCT for Healthcare Providers, consider the following steps:

**1** Determine which group(s) you are bringing CBCT for Healthcare Providers to.

**2** For each group, determine which offering makes the most sense to start with (the full course or one of the introductory offerings).

**3** Choose an Emory-certified CBCT teacher to facilitate the experience.

**4** Determine the format of the training (meeting frequency, length of sessions, online or in-person, etc.).

**5** Identify the date(s) and time(s) the training will take place.

## Implementation in Healthcare Education

Compassion training cannot be a mere desirable in healthcare education. Too many lives of healthcare professionals, residents, and students have been lost, and too many students have let the altruistic aspirations that led them to the pursuit of a noble career in healthcare succumb to cynicism and indifference. We can't afford to wait any longer.

Interactions with patients can either foster wellbeing or distress and burnout. Given the number of interactions that healthcare providers have with patients each day, the potential impact is significant, thus underscoring the importance of compassion and emotion-regulation education.

Communication skills, including awareness of non-verbal expressions and compassionate listening, are core to the art of medicine. The ability to be fully present, with mindful awareness of our unfolding emotions and body sensations as we listen and connect heart-to-heart with others, is an invaluable skill that needs to be developed.

## Bringing Compassion Training to Medical Education

Compassion must be integrated throughout the curriculum, in both pre-clinical and clinical years. This requires a decisive commitment by the leadership team to work toward implementation, which, with time and sustained diligence, should yield the cultural transformation. To succeed, the process needs to be all-inclusive and participatory. Following the steps described in Components 3 and 4, increasing levels of engagement will naturally occur, culminating in the full maturation and expression of the vision.

Ideally, Training Compassion for Healthcare Providers, the CBCT course offered on the digital learning platform, Compassion U, and facilitated by certified CBCT instructors/ambassadors, should be offered to first-year students. Then, preceptors in the clinical years need to take every opportunity to model compassionate care to their trainees. Ward rounds, sensitive conversations, communicating challenging news, and debriefing sessions are all invaluable opportunities for preceptors to model kind and compassionate care and to help students embody these skills.

## Bringing Compassion Training to Residency Programs

Residency training presents many challenges and is often physically exhausting and emotionally draining. It is not uncommon for interns to experience imposter syndrome and for residents to burn out and struggle with depression and anxiety. Compassion training is critical to protecting their health and wellbeing. Program directors can ensure this by integrating compassion training into their curricula and protecting training time from being infringed upon. Importantly, as underscored before, modeling compassion for their trainees is key.

# Component 4
## Support Ongoing Integration

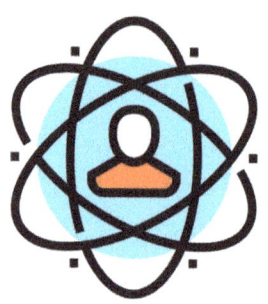

**4** **Support Ongoing Integration**

Sustain, develop, and continuously integrate CBCT for Healthcare Providers.

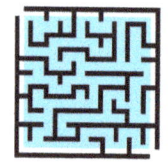 **Working through Barriers**

 **Monitoring and Adapting**

 **Sustaining a Culture of Compassion**

 **Encouraging Continued Practice**

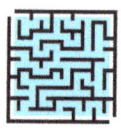 ## Working through Barriers

Lack of time and sense of urgency; the illusion that, once structural burdens are eliminated, wellbeing will spontaneously be realized; misconceptions about CBCT or not seeing value in compassion training—all these roadblocks (and others) can be overcome through education and training.

The process to overcome these roadblocks needs to be adaptable, comprehensive, and participatory. It should start with listening sessions to make stakeholders' needs and aspirations heard, identify what matters to them and what stands in the way, and what would motivate people to undertake the work of compassion training.

Healthcare providers are extremely busy, and the thought of adding an activity to an already very long day feels overwhelming—justifiably so. Often enough, they are already compromising precious time with family and friends to take care of patients.

However, once CBCT skills and insights become more embodied and compassion spontaneously arises in interactions with patients and colleagues, the sense that CBCT will take away time they don't have starts to disappear. Very brief interactions, when permeated with kindness and compassion, can make a significant difference for patients.

This section highlights some of the key barriers to the implementation process and offers guidance on how to address and work through them.

## Time

▶ There is inevitably time pressure in any organization. Prioritization, visible senior support, and long-term planning are key to finding the time for CBCT training. Another successful way to address the issue of time is to deliver the training in bite-sized periods of time; facilitating a 10-minute presentation can lead to interest in a 1-hour session, which may then lead to a half-day workshop.

## Money

▶ All organizations have finite financial resources and must allocate these accordingly. The cost of CBCT is relatively low and best viewed as an investment in the wellbeing of employees and the organization more widely.

## Buy-in

▶ Many organizations have effectively implemented CBCT for Healthcare Providers by first offering training to those who show an active interest, even if they make up a very small group. Once this group reports on their experiences and shares the benefits of the training with others in the community, the implementation can build on this initial success.

▶ Buy-in is also directly related to an effective communication plan. Helping the organization to understand the benefits and value-add proposition for them, personally and professionally, is critical. Reflecting the experience and feedback from CBCT participants within the organization will go a long way in building credibility, fostering authentic engagement, and promoting overall buy-in.

## Communication Issues

▶ Change initiatives often falter because the organization fails to provide consistent and ongoing communication about a prioritized initiative. Through multiple forms and iterations of communication, senior leaders must voice and message the impact, benefits, and progression of CBCT integration and training throughout the organization.

## Competing needs

▶ Many initiatives exist within every organization. CBCT for Healthcare Providers' ability to be overtly linked and aligned with the overall organizational strategy and subsequent initiatives is critical to the success of the overall implementation.

## Leadership and staff transition

▶ Leadership and staff turnover are inevitable in any organization. Establishing a culture and climate characterized by resilience, awareness, and compassion will ensure that the transition of key employees does not undermine efforts to further CBCT for Healthcare Providers training and integration.

 ## Monitoring and Adapting

CBCT ambassadors will play an important role in monitoring and adapting the implementation process over time. They will be responsible for engaging in periodic assessments to monitor the effectiveness of the CBCT for Healthcare Providers implementation. A comprehensive assessment might include examining providers' job satisfaction and overall wellbeing; incidences of burnout, imposter syndrome, and "quiet quitting"; incivility among members of the healthcare workforce; overt discrimination on the basis of gender, race, ethnicity, sexual identification, or faith tradition or lack thereof; aggressions and microaggressions; staff turnover rate; medical errors and malpractice lawsuits; readmission rates and recurring visits to the emergency room; provider suicide; and patients' satisfaction, compliance, clinical outcomes, and incivility toward medical staff, as just a few examples. Based on the results of the assessment, the ambassadors can determine if and how to adapt the process to improve outcomes.

CBCT ambassadors will also be responsible for leading "listen and learn" sessions periodically to monitor the progress of training in their respective teams or groups and assess whether there is a need to make any changes. They will then report their findings, maintaining participant anonymity, to their fellow ambassadors. This will facilitate a system-wide coordination of training progress and provide clarity as to the status of implementation and an all-inclusive culture of compassion. Since there will be a CBCT ambassador that is also a member of the leadership and C-suite, there will always be a direct line of communication to the leadership. This will enable simultaneous top-down and bottom-up coordinated actions to address emerging challenges and opportunities.

 ## Sustaining a Culture of Compassion

If we want to have a bountiful garden that produces a large harvest or many flowers, year after year, we need to tend to it with care. Likewise, with training, compassion naturally arises, but just like a bountiful garden, compassion needs to be tended to to remain flourishing. That is why it is so important, for the long-term sustainability of the culture of compassion and the wellbeing of all members of the healthcare workforce, that there will be ongoing opportunities to engage in their formal and informal CBCT practices. A meditation room for daily drop-in practice, a weekly session guided by a CBCT ambassador who is also a certified CBCT teacher, workshops, an annual retreat opportunity—these are all invaluable to ensure sustainability. In offering these opportunities, the leadership is also showing how much that culture of compassion means to them and to the system at large.

## Formal and Informal Practices

The CBCT for Healthcare Providers course offers two types of practices: formal and informal. Formal practices, otherwise known as meditations, are designed to strengthen particular skills or insights. Informal practices are ways we intentionally engage these skills and insights in our daily lives.

- Formal practices ("meditations"): mental exercises aimed at strengthening a particular skill or insight.

- Informal practices: ways to engage and apply CBCT skills and insights in our daily lives.

Informal practices differ from formal practices in that they are meant to be used right there and then, on the job, to foster emotion regulation and compassion in action, for the self and for others.

## Hiring and Onboarding Staff through the Lens of Compassion

As underscored throughout this guide, the vision is for sustaining a culture in which compassion is embedded throughout every part of the system, and the hiring process represents an invaluable opportunity to put that into practice. The job posting, the interviews, and the selection criteria should all be guided by this compassionate vision.

As part of the onboarding process, new employees should be offered the same orientation and informational session described in Component 2, to introduce them to the culture of compassion that guides the system. This way, every employee will get an overview of CBCT for Healthcare Providers and be invited to share in the vision of embedding compassion in every part of the system.

The program's ultimate success will be when the culture becomes known outside of the organization, and people will start applying for jobs enticed by its vision. These employees will feel proud and grateful to work for the system.

 # Encouraging Continued Practice

## Offer Community Practice Sessions

An important role of the CBCT ambassadors who have completed CBCT Teacher Certification, is leading weekly sessions with their team members. These sessions are essential to ensuring the sustainability of the skills they developed during the formal training.

These sessions provide the opportunity to revisit and/or reinforce key CBCT concepts and the Enduring Capabilities taught in the course. These sessions also represent an opportunity for the CBCT ambassador and facilitator to listen and learn about any challenges or opportunities that may have arisen within their team over the previous week, which can be shared with the fellow ambassadors as needed.

> These hour-long community practice sessions may include:
>
> - a guided meditation
> - an insight activity
> - an opportunity to share ongoing experiences with formal and informal practices
> - an exploration of new informal practices to bring into daily work

## Provide a Physical Space

A meditation room should be available for weekly community practice sessions and daily practice. This room should be a quiet place where everyone feels welcome, safe, and supported. Ideally, the room should be equipped to allow for these sessions to be made available in a hybrid virtual and in-person format to maximize participation. If this is not possible, practice sessions may be exclusively virtual.

## Encourage Bringing Informal Practices into Patient Care

Informal practices can be seamlessly integrated into patient care without requiring any extra time. These practices can promote grounding, non-judgmental awareness of one's physical and emotional state, relaxation, self-compassion, and connection with the intention to offer compassionate care. The community practice sessions are a great opportunity to encourage providers to continue integrating the skills and insights from the course into their daily life. The following are some examples of informal practices that may be integrated into daily patient care activities:

### Grounding

- **While washing hands:** Bring awareness to any sensations at the hand: The feeling of the hands rubbing one another, the temperature of the water, the soap, any foam, the contact with the paper towel drying the hands, and pausing for a moment to feel the two hands holding each other as a gesture of support and strength, an expression of self-compassion.

- **Before entering a patient's room:** Let awareness descend all the way down to the soles of the feet, and feel grounded, noticing the sensations of contact, temperature, and pressure, and pausing for a moment to set an intention to leave a footprint of kindness at each step.

- **While seated:** Take a moment to feel the sensations of bodily contact with the chair, perhaps warmth or pressure, and attune to the felt experience of being held and supported by the chair, anchored, grounded. It is safe to let the body relax and succumb to gravity.

### Mindful Listening

- **While listening to a patient:** Stay fully present, noticing the arousal of any sensations in the body such as tightness or contraction, being aware of tone of voice, body language, and facial expression, relaxing the muscles, and wholeheartedly listening, making the patient feel truly heard. How often are we thinking of a response to give while the patient is still talking? How often are we aware of how what we are hearing is making us feel in the body?

### Compassion with Equanimity

- **When facing challenges:** Remain mindful that we are humans, not superhumans, and that we may not have the power to control all the factors that may contribute to a patient's outcome, even though we so badly wish that we could. While recognizing that, set an intention to do what may be possible to help, irrespective of any outcome. Focus on the intention and the purpose we bring to it rather than on an outcome we cannot control.

### Bringing Meaning to Every Patient Encounter

1. **Ground:** Before entering a patient's rom, bring awareness to the soles of the feet, feeling grounded and supported.

2. **Check in:** Let awareness scan the body, noticing any tightness or contraction, particularly in the face, and letting the muscles relax with two deep breaths and slow exhalations.

3. **Bring awareness to the patient:** Begin to bring mindfulness to the patient that is in the room before you, attuning to their suffering, fears, anxieties, life circumstances, and how it might feel to be in that condition and see the world through their lenses. Attune to our shared human condition, and how that patient, just like you, wants to be healthy, safe, happy, loved, and live with ease, not to suffer.

4. **Connect with the motivation to help:** Notice feelings of affective empathy arising and let that be a reminder that, unlike that patient, we can do something to help, to make them feel more comfortable and cared for, even if all that may be possible is simply to hold their hand and offer a kind and supportive presence for a moment. Set an intention to bring kindness and compassion to that patient.

5. **Tap into compassion:** Open the door and greet the patient, remaining mindful of their suffering and of your intention to offer kind and compassionate care, without any expectation of reciprocity, as that patient may simply not be able to reciprocate our kindness. They may be in despair, perhaps feeling angry, neglected, abandoned, or discriminated against. Imagine a soothing and warm light radiating out of our chest, bringing some degree of healing and comfort to the patient.

6. **Offer kindness when leaving:** After performing whatever medical procedure is necessary, hold their hand as an expression of warm-heartedness before leaving the room.

7. **Self-regulate:** While stepping out the door, pause for a moment to check in with yourself, noticing sensations in your body and bringing the ease of a slow exhale to release and relax any tightness or tension.

8. **Attune to feelings of reward:** Attune to feelings of joy and reward for having left an imprint of kindness in that patient's life, and for having offered kind and compassionate care.

9. **Connect with gratitude:** Attune to the experience of gratitude for the opportunity to have been in a position to be of some help, to ease a bit of someone's suffering, and to make them feel genuinely cared for. Be grateful to the patient for giving you their trust and the opportunity to bring meaning to our livelihood.

10. **Sustain feelings of connection:** Proceed to the next patient encounter with feelings of connectedness, joy, reward, and purpose.

# Conclusion

The world is awakening to the need for compassion in all sectors, and in healthcare in particular. By infusing their healthcare systems with compassion, providers reconnect with their original motivation to work in this field and the sense of purpose associated with that. They cultivate more meaningful relationships with their colleagues and patients, and are more able to manage the ups and downs associated with this work. They renew their feelings of self-agency. The implementation of CBCT for Healthcare Providers serves healthcare workers, patients, families, and all those who interact with healthcare systems. It even contributes to the financial success of the systems that adopt it. The benefits of cultivating a sustainable culture of compassion in healthcare are endless. As Asch and colleagues underscored, "If kindness were a drug, the FDA would approve it."[13]

In this guide, we have outlined a step-by-step process for implementing CBCT for Healthcare Providers into a healthcare system. This process is a realistic approach, based on institutional experiences and best practices within healthcare, while allowing for individual variation and adaptation. How CBCT for Healthcare Providers is implemented will need to be continuously and creatively considered to encourage each system's buy-in, commitment, and sustained engagement.

For those who embark on this meaningful journey, know that the Emory Compassion Center will be there to support you, and that there is a growing network of others across the world—hospitals, clinics, educational institutions, corporate organizations, governmental and non-governmental bodies, researchers, and many others—who are pioneers in the field of compassion. As this network grows, the potential of each individual organization to make a difference will also grow, and each individual voice will be amplified. With sustained effort and mutual support, and with humility and self-compassion, this community will contribute to a more compassionate and ethical world for all.

**Keep In Touch**

**Visit:**
*compassionu. app/ for-organizations*

**Email:**
*partnerships. cbct@emory.edu*

# Notes

1   Howick, J., Dudko, M., Feng, S. N., Ahmed, A. A., Alluri, N., Nockels, K., Winter, R., & Holland, R. (2023). Why might medical student empathy change throughout medical school? A systematic review and thematic synthesis of qualitative studies. *BMC Medical Education,* 23(1), 270. https://doi.org/10.1186/s12909-023-04165-9; Kachel, T., Huber, A., Strecker, C., Höge, T., & Höfer, S. (2020). Development of cynicism in medical students: Exploring the role of signature character strengths and well-being. *Frontiers in Psychology*, 11, 328. https://doi.org/10.3389/fpsyg.2020.00328, Spányik, A., Simon, D., Rigó, A., Gács, B., Faubl, N., Füzesi, Z., Griffiths, M. D., & Demetrovics, Z. (2025). Cynicism among medical students: An in-depth analysis of mental health dynamics and protective factors in medical education using structural equation modeling. *PloS One*, 20(4), e0321274. https://doi.org/10.1371/journal.pone.0321274

2   Jain, L., Sarfraz, Z., Karlapati, S., Kazmi, S., Nasir, M. J., Atiq, N., Ansari, D., Shah, D., Aamir, U., Zaidi, K., Shakil Zubair, A., & Jyotsana, P. (2024). Suicide in healthcare workers: An umbrella review of prevalence, causes, and preventive strategies. *Journal of Primary Care & Community Health*, 15, 21501319241273242. https://doi.org/10.1177/21501319241273242; Nguyen, N., Spooner, E., O'Balle, P., Ashraf, H., Heskett, K., Zisook, S., & Davidson, J. E. (2025). The relationship between depression, burnout, and suicide among healthcare professionals: A scoping review. *Worldviews on Evidence-Based Nursing*, 22(3), e70037. https://doi.org/10.1111/wvn.70037; Rátiva Hernández, N. K., Carrero-Barragán, T.Y., Ardila, A. F., Rodríguez-Salazar, J. D., Lozada-Martinez, I. D.,Velez-Jaramillo, E., Ortega Delgado, D. A., Fiorillo Moreno, O., & Navarro Quiroz, E. (2023). Factors associated with suicide in physicians: A silent stigma and public health problem that has not been studied in depth. *Frontiers in Psychiatry*, 14, 1222972. https://doi.org/10.3389/fpsyt.2023.1222972; Shanafelt, T. D., Dyrbye, L. N., Sinsky, C., Trockel, M., Makowski, M. S., Tutty, M., Wang, H., Carlasare, L. E., & West, C. P. (2022). Imposter phenomenon in US physicians relative to the US working population. *Mayo Clinic Proceedings*, 97(11), 1981–1993. https://doi.org/10.1016/j.mayocp.2022.06.021; West, C. P., Dyrbye, L. N., & Shanafelt, T. D. (2018). Physician burnout: Contributors, consequences and solutions. *Journal of Internal Medicine*, 283(6), 516–529. https://doi.org/10.1111/joim.12752.

3   Fujii, C., & Iwasa, Y. Implications of nursing peer violence on patient safety: An integrative review. *International Nursing Review*, 72(3), e70042. https://doi.org/10.1111/inr.70042

4   Humphries, N., Morgan, K., Conry, M. C., McGowan, Y., Montgomery, A., & McGee, H. (2014). Quality of care and health professional burnout: narrative literature review. *International Journal of Health Care Quality Assurance*, 27(4), 293–307. https://doi.org/10.1108/IJHCQA-08-2012-0087

5   Rathert, C., Mittler, J. N., Vogus, T. J., & Lee, Y. S. H. (2023). Better outcomes through patient - Provider therapeutic connections? An exploratory study of proposed

mediating variables. *Social Science & Medicine* (1982), 338, 116290. https://doi.org/10.1016/j.socscimed.2023.116290

6   Trzeciak, S., & Mazzarelli, A. (2019). *Compassionomics: The Revolutionary Scientific Evidence that Caring Makes a Difference.* Pensacola, FL: Studer Group.

7   Ash, M., Harrison, T., Pinto, M., DiClemente, R., & Negi, L. T. (2021). A model for cognitively-based compassion training: Theoretical underpinnings and proposed mechanisms. *Social Theory & Health*, 19, 43–67 (2021).

8   Ash, M. J., Walker, E. R., DiClemente, R. J., Florian, M. P., Palmer, P. K., Wehrmeyer, K., Negi, L. T., Grant, G. H., Raison, C. L., & Mascaro, J. S. (2021). Compassion meditation training for hospital chaplain residents: A pilot study. *Journal of Health Care Chaplaincy*, 27(4), 191–206. https://doi.org/10.1080/08854726.2020.1723189 ; Mascaro, J. S., Rilling, J. K., Tenzin Negi, L., & Raison, C. L. (2013). Compassion meditation enhances empathic accuracy and related neural activity. *Social Cognitive and Affective Neuroscience*, 8(1), 48–55. https://doi.org/10.1093/scan/nss095; Mascaro, J. S., Kelley, S., Darcher, A., Negi, L. T., Worthman, C., Miller, A., & Raison, C. (2016). Meditation buffers medical student compassion from the deleterious effects of depression. *Journal of Positive Psychology*, 13(2), 133–142. https://doi.org/10.1080/17439760.2016.1233348; Mascaro, J. S., Palmer, P. K., Willson, M., Ash, M. J., Florian, M. P., Srivastava, M., Sharma, A., Jarrell, B., Walker, E. R., Kaplan, D. M., Palitsky, R., Cole, S. P., Grant, G. H., & Raison, C. L. (2023). The language of compassion: Hospital chaplains' compassion capacity reduces patient depression via other-oriented, inclusive language. *Mindfulness*, 14(10), 2485–2498. https://doi.org/10.1007/s12671-022-01907-6; Mascaro, J. S., Palmer, P. K., Ash, M. J., Florian, M. P., Kaplan, D. M., Palitsky, R., Cole, S. P., Shelton, M., Raison, C. L., & Grant, G. H. (2025). A randomized controlled trial of a compassion-centered spiritual health intervention to improve hospital inpatient outcomes. *PloS One, 20*(3), e0313602. https://doi.org/10.1371/journal.pone.0313602; Pace, T. W. W., Negi, L. T., Adame, D. D., Cole, S. P., Sivilli, T. I., Brown, T. D., Issa, M. J., & Raison, C. L. (2009). Effect of compassion meditation on neuroendocrine, innate immune and behavioral responses to psychosocial stress. *Psychoneuroendocrinology*, 34(1), 87–98. https://doi.org/10.1016/j.psyneuen.2008.08.011

9   Pace, T. W. W. et al. (2009);; Pace, T., Negi, L., Donaldson-Lavelle, B., Ozawa-de Silva, B., Reddy, S., Cole, S., Craighead, L., & Raison, C. (2012). Cognitively-Based Compassion Training reduces peripheral inflammation in adolescents in foster care with high rates of early life adversity. *BMC Complementary and Alternative Medicine*, 12(Suppl 1), 175. https://doi.org/10.1186%2F1472-6882-12-S1-P175; Pace, T. W. W., Negi, L. T., Dodson-Lavelle, B., Ozawa-de Silva, B., Reddy, S. D., Cole, S. P., Danese, A., Craighead, L. W., & Raison, C. L. (2013). Engagement with Cognitively-Based Compassion Training is associated with reduced salivary C-reactive protein from before to after training in foster care program adolescents. *Psychoneuroendocrinology*, 38(2), 294–299. https://doi.org/10.1016/j.psyneuen.2012.05.019; Reddy, S., Negi, L., Dodson-Lavelle, B., Ozawa-de Silva, B., Pace, T., Cole, S., Raison, C., & Craighead, L. (2013). Cognitive-based compassion training: A promising prevention strategy for at-risk adolescents. *Journal of Child and Family Studies*, 22(2), 219–230. http://dx.doi.org/10.1007/s10826-012-9571-7; Titanji, B. K., Tejani, M., Farber, E. W., Mehta, C. C., Pace, T. W., Meagley, K., Gavegnano, C., Harrison, T., Kokubun, C. W., Negi, S. D., Schinazi, R. F., & Marconi, V. C. (2022). Cognitively Based Compassion Training

for HIV immune nonresponders—An attention-placebo randomized controlled trial. *Journal of Acquired Immune Deficiency Syndromes*, 89(3), 340–348. https://doi.org/10.1097/QAI.0000000000002874.

10  Lang, A. J., Casmar, P., Hurst, S., Harrison, T., Golshan, S., Good, R., Essex, M., & Negi, L. (2017). Compassion meditation for veterans with posttraumatic stress disorder (PTSD): A nonrandomized study. *Mindfulness*, 11(1), 63–74. https://doi.org/10.1007/s12671-017-0866-z; Mascaro, J. S., Kelley, S., Darcher, A., Negi, L. T., Worthman, C., Miller, A., & Raison, C. (2016). Meditation buffers medical student compassion from the deleterious effects of depression. *Journal of Positive Psychology*, 13(2), 133–142. https://doi.org/10.1080/17439760.2016.1233348..

11  Mascaro, J. S. et al. (2016).

12  Lang, A. J. et al. (2017).

13  Reddy, S. et al. (2013).

14  Desbordes, G., Negi, L. T., Pace, T. W., Wallace, B. A., Raison, C. L., & Schwartz. E. L. (2012). Effects of mindful-attention and compassion meditation training on amygdala response to emotional stimuli in an ordinary, non-meditative state. *Frontiers in Human Neuroscience*, 6, 292. https://doi.org/10.3389/fnhum.2012.00292; Mascaro, J. S. et al. (2016).

15  Mascaro, J., Rilling, J., Negi, L. T., & Raison, C. (2012). Compassion meditation enhances empathic accuracy and related neural activity. *Social Cognitive and Affective Neuroscience*, 8(1), 48–55. https://doi.org/10.1093/scan/nss095

16  Gonzalez-Hernandez, E., Romero, R., Campos, D., Burychka, D., Diego-Pedro, R., Baños, R., Negi, L., & Cebolla, A. (2018). Cognitively-Based Compassion Training (CBCT) in breast cancer survivors: A randomized clinical trial study. *Integrative Cancer Therapies*, 17(3), 684–696. https://doi.org/10.1177/1534735418772095; Sun, S., Pickover, A. M., Goldberg, S. B., Bhimji, J., Nguyen, J. K., Evans, A. E., Patterson, B., & Kaslow, N. J. (2019). For whom does Cognitively Based Compassion Training (CBCT) work? An analysis of predictors and moderators among African American suicide attempters. *Mindfulness*, 10(11), 2327–2340. https:// doi.org/10.1007/s12671-019-01207-6; Titanji, B. K. et al. (2022).

17  Behan, C., & Kelly, B. (2025). *Handbook of Compassion in Healthcare: A Practical Approach* (pp. 52–59). Cambridge: Cambridge University Press.

18  Trzeciak, S., & Mazzarelli, A. (2019). *Compassionomics: The Revolutionary Scientific Evidence That Caring Makes a Difference*. Pensacola, FL: Studer Group. Mascaro, J. S. et al. (2025).

19  Ahmed, Z., Ellahham, S., Soomro, M., Shams, S., & Latif, K. (2024). Exploring the impact of compassion and leadership on patient safety and quality in healthcare systems: A narrative review. BMJ *Open Quality*, 13(Suppl 2), e002651. https://doi.org/10.1136/bmjoq-2023-002651

20  Trzeciak, S., & Mazzarelli, A. (2019).

21  Redelmeier, D. A., Molin, J. P., & Tibshirani, R. J. (1995). A randomised trial of compassionate care for the homeless in an emergency department. *Lancet*, 345(8958), 1131–1134. https://doi.org/10.1016/s0140-6736(95)90975-3

22  Holzer, K. J., Bollepalli, H., Carron, J., Yaeger, L. H., Avidan, M. S., Lenze, E. J., & Abraham, J. (2024). The impact of compassion-based interventions on perioperative anxiety and depression: A systematic review and meta-analysis. *Journal of Affective Disorders*, 365, 476–491. https://doi.org/10.1016/j.jad.2024.08.110

23  Barton, M. F., Groves, J., Guevel, B., Saint, K., Barton, B. L., Hamza, M., & Papatheodorou, S. I. (2023). Mindfulness-based interventions for the reduction of postoperative pain in hip and knee arthroplasty patients: A systematic review and meta-analysis. *Cureus*, 15(6), e40102. https://doi.org/10.7759/cureus.40102

24  Tung, K. M., Su, Y., Kang, Y. N., Hou, W. H., Hoang, K. D., Chen, K. H., & Chen, C. (2024). Effects of mindfulness-based preoperative intervention for patients undergoing elective surgery: A meta-analysis. *Journal of Psychosomatic Research*, 181, 111666. https://doi.org/10.1016/j.jpsychores.2024.111666

25  Wang, X., Lu, Y., Gu, C., Shao, J., Yan, Y., & Zhang, J. (2024). Mindfulness meditation reduces stress and hospital stay in gastrointestinal tumor patients during perioperative period. *Medical Science Monitor: International Medical Journal of Experimental and Clinical Research*, 30, e945834. https://doi.org/10.12659/MSM.945834

26  WHO Special Programme on Primary Health Care. (2025). *Compassion and Primary Health Care*. https://www.who.int/publications/i/item/9789240105249

27  Dyrbye, L. N., Brushaber, D. E., & West, C. P. (2024). Reports of burnout among historically marginalized and female graduating medical students during the COVID-19 pandemic. *Academic Medicine: Journal of the Association of American Medical Colleges*, 99(12), 1385–1395. https://doi.org/10.1097/ACM.0000000000005854; Fadum, E. A., Ekeberg, Ø., & Hem, E. (2025). Job satisfaction in doctors with suicidal ideation: a national longitudinal panel study 2002–2021. *BMC Psychiatry*, 25(1), 666. https://doi.org/10.1186/s12888-025-07101-x; Hashem, Z., & Zeinoun, P. (2020). Self-compassion explains less burnout among healthcare professionals. *Mindfulness*, 11(11), 2542–2551. https://doi.org/10.1007/s12671-020-01469-5; Iserson, K. (2024). From magical thinking to suicide: Understanding emergency physicians' psychological struggle. *The American Journal of Emergency Medicine*, 78. https://doi.org/10.1016/j.ajem.2024.01.001; Jain, L. et al. (2024); Jung, E., & Jung, Y. E. (2025). The impact of self-compassion on enhancing the professional quality of life for healthcare workers. *Journal of Korean Medical Science*, 40(14), e141. https://doi.org/10.3346/jkms.2025.40.e141; Luong, J., Prasad, J., Huang, E. S., Hutter, J., McWatt, S., Brassett, C., Stearns, D., Sagoo, M. G., Bhugra, D., Noel, G., Molodynski, A., & Wu, A. (2025). The state of mental health in medical students in 2023 from 18 countries. *Academic Psychiatry: The Journal of the American Association of Directors of Psychiatric Residency Training and the Association for Academic Psychiatry*. Advance online publication. https://doi.org/10.1007/s40596-025-02143-5; Mezrich J. L. (2025). Alone in the dark: Medical malpractice stress syndrome and implications for radiologists. *AJR. American Journal of Roentgenology*. Advance online publication. https://doi.org/10.2214/AJR.25.33290; Nguyen, N. et al. (2025).; Rátiva Hernández, N. K. et al. (2023); Shanafelt, T. D. et al. (2022); Thakur, S., Chauhan, V., Galwankar, S., Lateef, F., Daniel, P., Cakir, Z., Lugo, K. M., Basnet, S., Bildik, B., Azahaf, S., Vural, S., Difyeli, B. H., & Moreno-Walton, L. (2025). Gender disparities and burnout among emergency physicians: A systematic review by the World Academic Council of Emergency Medicine-Female Leadership Academy for Medical Excellence. *The Western Journal of Emergency Medicine*, 26(2), 338–346. https://doi.org/10.5811/westjem.29331

28  Klotz, A. C., & Bolino, M. C. (2022). When quiet quitting is worse than the real thing. *Harvard Business Review*. https://hbr.org/2022/09/when-quiet-quitting-is-worse-than-the-real-thing

29  Ng, I. K., Goh, W. G., Thong, C., & Teo, K. S. (2025). 'Quiet quitting' among medical practitioners: a hallmark of burnout, disillusionment and cynicism. *Journal of the Royal Society of Medicine*, 118(3), 73–77. https://doi.org/10.1177/01410768241311059; Scheyett A. (2022). Quiet quitting. Social Work, 68(1), 5–7. https://doi.org/10.1093/sw/swac051

30  West, C. P. et al. (2018).

31  Waltz, M., Cadigan, R. J., Joyner, B., Ossman, P., & Davis, A. (2019). Perils of the hidden curriculum: Emotional labor and "bad" pediatric proxies. *The Journal of Clinical Ethics*, 30(2), 154–162.

32  Kerasidou, A., & Horn, R. (2016). Making space for empathy: Supporting doctors in the emotional labour of clinical care. *BMC Medical Ethics*, 17, 8. https://doi.org/10.1186/s12910-016-0091-7

33  Thangarasu, S., Renganathan, G., & Natarajan, P. (2021). Empathy can be taught, and patients teach it best. *Journal of Medical Education and Curricular Development*, 8, 23821205211000346. https://doi.org/10.1177/23821205211000346

34  Chwyl, C., Chen, P., & Zaki, J. (2021). Beliefs about self-compassion: Implications for coping and self-improvement. Personality & Social Psychology Bulletin, 47(9), 1327–1342. https://doi.org/10.1177/0146167220965303; Germer, C., & Neff, K. (2019). *Teaching the Mindful Self-Compassion Program: A Guide for Professionals*. New York: The Guilford Press.

35  Breines, J. G., & Chen, S. (2012). Self-compassion increases self-improvement motivation. *Personality & Social Psychology Bulletin*, 38(9), 1133–1143. https://doi.org/10.1177/0146167212445599

36  Chwyl, C. et al. (2021).

37  Kirschner, H., Kuyken, W., Wright, K., Roberts, H., Brejcha, C., & Karl, A. (2019). Soothing your heart and feeling connected: A new experimental paradigm to study the benefits of self-compassion. *Clinical Psychological Science: A Journal of the Association for Psychological Science*, 7(3), 545–565. https://doi.org/10.1177/2167702618812438).

www.ingramcontent.com/pod-product-compliance
Lightning Source LLC
Chambersburg PA
CBHW041126120626
46547CB00019B/2871